FUNCTIONAL STRENGTH

THE KEY TO PAIN-FREE MOVEMENT

This publication is designed to provide competent and reliable information regarding the subject matter covered. However, it should not be substituted for the advice of a physician. Always consult your physician prior to participating in any exercise program. The author and publisher specifically disclaim any liability that is incurred from the use or application of the contents of this book.

10 digit ISBN 1-4392-0495-0
13 digit ISBN 978-1-4392-0495-5

FUNCTIONAL STRENGTH
THE KEY TO PAIN-FREE MOVEMENT

BY CHRIS JANKE

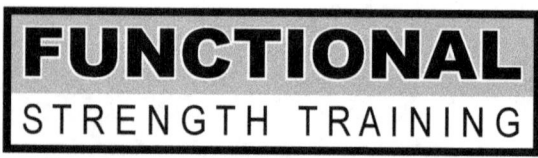

FUNCTIONAL
STRENGTH TRAINING
Posture • Fitness • Athletics

At Functional Strength Training, we are committed to empowering people to make profound changes in their lives. We believe that one of the greatest ways to enhance your overall health is to improve your posture and functional strength.

My intention in writing this book is to provide you with another option. I want to introduce you to a way of thinking about exercise that has changed my life and the lives of many others.

I dedicate this book to all of my clients: past, present, and future. Every day, I see evidence of how amazing the human body is, much more intelligent in its design than the most state-of-the-art piece of equipment in any gym.

408.509.3497
www.FSTworkout.com

FUNCTIONAL STRENGTH
THE KEY TO PAIN-FREE MOVEMENT

CONTENTS:

INTRODUCTION

MY STORY

When I was young I was like any other kid. In elementary school, I remember being in class, squirming in my chair. My eyes were glued to the clock, which seemed to slow down the closer it got to recess. Finally, the second hand would brush past the 12 and the bell would ring, and we knew that it was time to play. At that point, it was a mad dash to the playground. I couldn't get there fast enough. Tetherball, 4-square, handball, basketball, we always had enough to do. I remember having no trouble making up games to play, and all of them involved running, jumping, or climbing on something. Recess was twenty minutes, which would pass by in a flash. I remember feeling that time flies when you're having fun. Twenty minutes into recess, the warning bell rang. After that first bell, we still had five minutes left to get to class. Every kid knew exactly how long it took to sprint back to class and make it into his or her seat before the second bell sounded five minutes later. It took me less than a minute to get to my seat, so I had about four extra minutes of recess, which was of course my favorite subject in school. We would all return to class in a sprint, still panting after we had taken our seats. The teacher would begin talking, and we'd all think about what we would be doing when the lunch bell rang.

After school hours it was more of the same. I loved sports, and loved playing with friends. I have played sports for as long as I can remember. As a six-year-old, I played baseball and soccer. A few years later, I began playing basketball. When I was 10, the San Jose Sharks became the newest team in the NHL, so my friends and I started playing street hockey. There was always a sport in season. In the spring and summer, baseball filled our schedules. As fall approached and school began, it was all soccer. There were basketball leagues just after that. On the rare weekend when we weren't in an organized sport, we would walk to the park and throw the football around. Sometimes after school, my dad, brother, and I would play catch in the front yard. My life revolved around movement, and I loved every minute of it.

As I approached my teenage years, sports became more competitive. As this happened, I began to gravitate toward basketball. Like most of my friends, I had dreams of play-ing high school and then college basketball. In order to get stronger, everyone was lifting weights, so naturally I wanted to also. I remember, even as a ten-year-old, nag-ging my dad to take me to the gym to lift. I wanted to get buff. Finally, when I turned 14, I was allowed to work out with weights at the local gym. A staff member gave me an orientation, and then my dad and I were allowed to use the equipment. This was a great way to bond with my dad, and allowed us to get stronger and fitter together.

I stayed active throughout high school. I loved sports even more, especially basketball. In eighth grade my passion for basketball exploded and became an all-out obsession. All I wanted to do was play professional basketball in the NBA. All I would talk about with friends was basketball. There was no off-season. After our last basketball game of the school year, we would join recreation leagues. I would go to the local gym or park and work on my game. On warm summer days, I would go to the park with friends and practice. We would be there all day. Every day became very focused on basketball.

I was always very active and considered myself healthy. But when I was thirteen I had an experience that proved I wasn't as healthy as I thought. My first bout with severe lower back pain occurred when I was in eighth grade. I was warming up for basketball practice when I felt a "twinge" in my lower back, which I had never felt before. It wasn't particularly bad so I played through it. But it only got worse as I kept playing. Certain motions would flare it up again. When this happened I would just sit out for a minute and go back in. Finally, I had to come out for good because my back went into an all-out spasm. Sitting on the sidelines, I kept massaging my back to get the spasm to go away. I wanted to get back onto the court. Then my coach said something that I know I will never forget. His words stay with me to this day: "once you've injured it, there's nothing you can do but rest." I would not be going back in. Coach recommended that I have it checked out, so I did. X-Rays would show that I had a bulged disk. The space in between my lower two lumbar vertebrae was smaller than it was supposed to be. It was pinching on a nerve, which was causing my pain. I missed a week of practice, and then returned to the court when the sharp pain went away. I finished out the season without missing any more playing time, but I had to deal with constant soreness in my lower back. I now had a new way to bond with my dad: when we took trips to the chiropractor together.

The pain would only get worse. In high school, I suffered from sciatic pain shooting down my left leg. I actually cannot even call this pain; it's more of an absence of feeling altogether. The sciatic nerve runs through the pelvis and down the leg to the feet. If that gets pinched, it doesn't feel good. It affected every movement I tried to make. I could not bend forward to touch my toes anymore. In fact, I could barely get to my knees before my hamstrings started screaming at me. When I stretched it, I didn't get a feeling of a stretched muscle; I actually felt the nerve pinch even more. When I ran, my teammates told me that my left leg looked funny. They said I just "flung it" in front of me. The reason was that I couldn't control it because of the pinched nerve. With everything I did, I always felt that nerve. In fact, I could almost trace its path down my leg. Even though the pinch was in the hip, I could feel the pain in my hamstring, calf, and sometimes even in the foot. Despite these pains, I persisted in playing the sports that I loved. The injuries were not severe enough to keep me completely off of the court. I just played through the injuries, plus I was learning to live with them.

As a senior in high school, a friend of mine invited me to go water skiing with him. I was excited. I had never been water skiing before, and had never really been into water sports in general. His family had a house right on the river, and a boat parked on the dock. We took the 4-hour drive just after school ended on a Friday. After arriving, we unpacked our things and settled in. Saturday morning we started waterskiing early. I enjoyed being out in the water and the sun, but really did not pick up the water skiing very well. I had a difficult time getting into a standing position. Most of my day was spent gripping the handles as hard as I could and hoping that this would be the time I would stand and ride. But that time never came. I didn't get up to the surface all day. It was a little frustrating, but I felt content that I had given it a shot. After the day on the water, we headed back to the house to relax for the evening. We had a few hours to kill before dinner, so we sat on the couch to watch a movie. It was very odd, but about halfway through the movie I noticed that my head was beginning to tilt to the side. My neck started getting very tight, and I couldn't straighten up my head. By the end of the movie, my ear was almost at my shoulder and it hurt when I tried to move. I couldn't stand up. My friend's dad had to hold my head as he walked me to the car. In the car, every little bump sent electrical shocks into my neck. It was excruciating. I missed four days of school the next week, and was given the nickname of "old man."

Kids can be cruel. High school kids are no exception. And at an all-boys high school, it can feel a bit like you're in a locker room all day long. When I returned to school my new nickname was already there waiting for me. For the first half of my first day back, I got a good tease from all of my buddies. Once they got tired and the jokes got old, it died down a bit. But other people knew about the injury too. Of course all of my teammates and my coaches knew because I missed practices. I don't think that any of them had ever seen someone who missed almost a week of school because their neck was tight. I was quite the talk of the school. Even coaches were perplexed by my seemingly "old" body. It seemed that nobody at school had a problem voicing what they thought of my injury. I know that their intention was good, they were just trying to make jokes. But I cannot fully describe how embarrassing, annoying, and old those jokes got. Have you ever watched a video of a comedy show 200 times? The first time it may be hilarious. The next few times it's still funny but the suspense is gone. Watching that video any more just becomes torture, no matter how funny it was the first time. I had the privilege of hearing the same joke told at my expense by everyone I knew, and even some people that I didn't know. There is an emotional side of pain that has nothing to do with the initial injury, but it can hurt just as much.

The next year was my first year in college. It was also the next time I would experience crippling pain. One weekend, I went with a friend to her family barbecue. One of her uncles was an avid golfer, so he took us to the driving range to hit some balls while we waited for the food to cook. I have never been especially good at, or fond of, golf, but I love the driving range. I love smacking the golf ball as hard as I can and just watching how far it goes. After hitting a full bucket each, we went back to the barbecue. The food was almost ready, so I sat down to watch the football game that was on. Within 10 minutes the food was done, and everyone stood up and walked to the kitchen to make a plate. I stayed on the couch. Not because I don't like food, but because I literally couldn't move. This time it was my lower back. The spasm sent pain from my lower back up and down my body. It locked up so badly I couldn't get any movement out of it. I couldn't even stand up. For the next hour, I became the brunt of everyone's jokes, including my own. It's easier to make jokes than to try and be macho about it. I cannot fully describe how embarrassing it is to be 19-years-old and have two middle-aged men help me walk to the car. All I was thinking during that hobble to the car was that I should be helping them walk. And there it was, my reputation of "old man" was spreading. The worst part about that day was I didn't get any food.

I escaped any embarrassing incidents for the next couple years. I still had soreness more often than not, but nothing sharp or debilitating. The pain was more of a dull, constant tightness that I just learned to live with. I stopped moving as much, and then I started the college partying scene and getting involved in my schoolwork. I didn't really think much about sports, movement, or my back. I kind of stopped caring. Sometimes I would take an anti-inflammatory if it got too bad, but for the most part I stayed just out of the reach of pain.

All of that changed during my third year in college. I was working out heavily with weights. I would go to the gym every morning with two of my friends. These guys were very strong, and I was definitely out of my league. Despite my lack of strength, they took me under their wing and helped me to increase my bench press and other weight. The goal was to get up as much weight as possible and get big. To help us get big, we were taking creatine and protein after our workouts. After several months, we had all achieved our goal of getting big. I weighed 195 pounds (while I was playing sports in high school I weighed about 170 pounds). I was bulky, slow, and tight. I could barely touch my knees in a forward bend. Slowly, the pain in the back began to return. I had been without any big pains for two years, so I had forgotten what it was like to constantly live with it. I am still not sure what was different about this particular experience of pain, but for some reason I finally got fed up.

Our college gym was segregated: the weights for males, cardio and stretching for females. Occasionally you would see a female lifting weights or a male on the cardio machine, but it was rare. I set aside this bizarre gender segregation and put myself first. I was tired of being "the old man." I had all these goals that I wanted to achieve, yet some days I couldn't even get out of bed without limping. There comes a point when we see our lives from the outside. Looking at my life from an outsider's perspective I realized that I had given up. For so many years I lived with pain because that's what I thought I had to do. It never occurred to me that I could get out of it. It was never a reality to me. But now it was, and it was time to change. I told the guys that I would be taking a break from the weights for a while, and going to the girls' side to workout. For the next few months, I did a 90-minute daily stretching routine. Not knowing much about what I was doing, I did what felt good at the time. My basic plan was that if something was tight, I would stretch it. It helped a little. My pain was not gone, but I was able to touch my toes for the first time in years. This was my first glimpse that there might be a better way to exercise.

Even though I made the choice to change, pain would still be my constant companion. There was always a low-level discomfort that would occasionally turn into pain for a day or two and then resume its place as discomfort. It never really went away, but it lessened enough to where I could pursue basketball again. After I graduated college, I went into the same gym that my dad and I used to work out in, and I hired a personal trainer. This trainer was ahead of his time, and didn't use the traditional weights. We did a lot of balance work and core strengthening. I finally felt that I could try to live my dream, so I began to try out for semi-pro basketball teams. My conditioning was phenomenal. I was dunking a basketball with two hands; I was beating everyone up and down the court. Through all this, my back got a lot better, but the pain didn't go away. Once or twice a month I would have to cancel my training session because it just hurt too badly. Also, since I was playing more basketball and at a higher level, another injury kept appearing. I would sprain my ankle about once every three months. It was always the same ankle and in the same direction. These sprains would keep me off the court for a week or more. The podiatrist said I had flat feet, so he gave me arch supports to build up an arch. That didn't help. If anything, it made it worse because now it was like I was wearing high heels. So the ankles kept twisting. My training was intense, but it was never consistent because of the constant interruptions. What I kept asking myself was, "If I'm in such great shape, why do I keep getting hurt?" I couldn't understand it.

At this point, I was absolutely fed up with pain. I began to see every pain as a signal that something was wrong with how I used my body. It was my personal mission to learn everything that I could. The first thing I did was become a personal trainer. Soon after I got certified I got a job at the same gym where I would work out. Like my childhood days, my life revolved around movement. In the morning I would go to the gym to workout and work on my basketball skills. I would walk home for a quick snack, and later in the day I would return to the gym to do an intense work out. In the afternoon and evening I would work and see clients. Throughout these days I was constantly learning.

FUNCTIONAL STRENGTH

I felt like I was close to an answer. I was trying different modalities to see if there was a common thread that they had. I scheduled appointments with various practitioners doing different forms of bodywork. These sessions helped me with my pain, and allowed me some insight to help my clients, but my number one goal was to get myself out of pain.

My standards for myself went way up. I wouldn't accept even the slightest bit of pain anymore. I needed to eliminate it completely, but it was still lingering. I could still feel some residual pain from the past, which kept me looking for the key that would get me out of my pain permanently. It was a massage therapist who planted a seed in my head that started me thinking about posture. She was a co-worker at the time, and studying to practice massage therapy. I was a muscle-head personal trainer, complaining about my ankle. She took one look at me and said, "of course your ankle hurts, your whole body is leaning forward and your weight is on your toes. Your Achilles tendons are overworked. It's just a posture problem." Even though I was a personal trainer at this time, I had never thought of that before. You mean the position of my body is affecting my ankle pain? Could this be true of my back too? My previous paradigm was the same as my eighth grade basketball coach, "once it's injured, there's nothing you can do." Now I had hope. Posture made sense. Maybe all of my injuries were connected. Maybe if I balanced my body and worked on my posture, everything would just work itself out. The more I researched, the more I was convinced of the importance of posture. It was time to start out on a new path, but this time I knew that it was the right one.

That's when the real work began. Even after that spark

of insight, it would be another two years before I had the tools to do anything about my pain. Once I learned what I needed to learn, I got to it. The exercises took daily attention, but I did them. I had to start from scratch. I had to re-teach my body how to move. I went back to the days when movement was fun. Over the next few months, I felt like I was peeling back layers of an onion. After I uncovered one imbalance I would peel it off only to find another underneath. The entire experience was so inspiring. I could feel younger everyday. Movement became easier. When doing day-to-day tasks, there was a new gracefulness about me. I felt like I could once again control my movements. As I got more functional, I couldn't stop. I had to learn more so that I could pass it on. Functional strength has been my passion ever since.

This never would have happened if I didn't come to the point of being sick of my pain. It's important to know what to do, but then you have to do it. I had such a powerful reason why I wanted to get out of pain that all of the setbacks didn't stop me. The discipline to do these exercises daily was easy to find because I knew why I was doing them. I didn't just have an interest in getting rid of my pain, I was absolutely committed to doing whatever it took to be done with it. Without this mindset, I don't think I would have made it. I needed that burning desire inside of myself to restore my posture and function, to return to when I had no pain, and when movement felt good. Just getting to the point when I decided that I wasn't going to live in pain anymore took years. But once I made up my mind, there was no going back. The body quickly and easily walked the path that my mind had already carved, and the struggle became worth it. There was meaning to my pain, and there was hope that I would get rid of it.

FUNCTIONAL STRENGTH

I am now out of pain. I haven't sprained my ankle in over three years, and I now have arches in my feet (even without shoes) where I previously had none. My lower back has relaxed and my sciatic pain is gone. I can feel when my body gets out of position, and can correct it long before it manifests as pain. My athleticism has gone way up too. I have more control over my body than at any other time in my life. I have the benefit of adult strength combined with child-like flexibility. What a great feeling it is to be able to twist and turn on the basketball court without pain. It's a different kind of strength, and I feel even stronger than I did when I was lifting all that weight in college. I routinely run circles around "muscle heads" on the basketball court because they are too tight to move properly. I know what it's like to be stuck in that kind of body, since I was for so long. I am back to about the same weight I was in high school, which allows me the freedom to move without useless muscle weighing me down. I still lift weights, but it is with a new goal. My number one goal is to restore my posture and function. We are all meant to be functionally strong with good posture. It's the most natural I've felt since my early childhood.

I have a new paradigm now, that the body is capable of repairing itself if you just put it in the right position. Injuries are just ways that your body communicates with you. If you know how to listen, you can give the body what it needs. Now I try to help others to navigate the same path that I traveled, to teach them how to listen to their bodies. I have devoted myself to this career path because I am committed to helping other people correct their posture without having to experience what I did. I know what pain is. Sometimes I wish that I didn't, but then I realize that although the path was difficult, it was worth it (It's easy for me to say that when I'm not experiencing it now. If you asked me then if the pain was worth it I don't know if I could have responded positively.). Although it took me years before I found the solution, it's really not complicated. It is right under our noses. Function is so basic that if you told me about it as a six-year-old I would have understood it. It is what I innately understood as a kid when I was making up all of those games. I knew what healthy movement was. As I grew up I forgot how great it felt to just move freely. Pain kept me away from child-like movement for thirteen years, but I have it back. I feel like I did when I was a kid, playing on the playground and not wanting recess to end.

PART ONE

THE NEED FOR A PARADIGM SHIFT

THE TREADMILL OF HEALTH

"No pain, no gain." This short saying has defined the fitness industry for years. It refers to that "burn" that you get when working out, ensuring that you get the maximum gains possible. We beat up our bodies by pushing them to the absolute limit. Pain is seen as a good thing. It's a measuring stick to judge how hard you pushed. Many people don't feel like they worked out unless they feel sore the next day. Pain and movement have been paired together. We have come to see fitness as a painful endeavor. But what happens when these pains interfere with the activities that we enjoy most? Many people think that there is no other option except stopping these activities that bring so much joy to our lives. We blame old age, a past injury, or a host of other excuses as to why we're not able to participate in our favorite pastimes. We feel powerless to stop the grip of pain. So many people are stuck: we are told that we need to move and be active, but it hurts to move. What do we do? Unfortunately, "no pain, no gain" has worked its way into our collective consciousness. But we need to find a better way.

Although many gyms have become more high tech, the basic "no pain, no gain" paradigm has remained. If we want to solve the problem of painful workouts, we need to change the way we think about exercise. The mind-set of typical gym-goers is what I call the "Treadmill of Health." Much of the Treadmill of Health mentality is on "maximum output," meaning that the emphasis is on the maximum amount of "x" that you can do. This could be your maximum heart rate or your maximum bench press or a host of other "maximums." Whatever the test, it's about "maxing out." For example, when a body builder considers how much weight to do on their bench press, they will begin with their "maximum bench." This number is the maximum weight you can do in one repetition. Then they do a certain number of repetitions of a certain percentage of their max. The goal for weight lifters is to lift more and more weight. This goal is so prevalent in gyms today, that Saturday Night Live did a sketch on it, "What's your bench?" Callers would call into the radio show and ask fitness-related questions. The hosts of the show would ask them, "What's your bench?" When the hosts heard the puny number, they began laughing. "Ha ha ha, that's nothing. I can lift that with my little pinky finger." Even if the caller said that they benched 600 pounds, the hosts would still laugh. This skit was an exaggeration of an already-present mentality in gyms: more weight is better. It is a mentality that I was stuck in for so long. Looking back, I can see that during those times that I could lift the most weight, I did not feel better. Often, adding weight means experiencing more pain. When that became the case for me, I began looking for a better way.

The Treadmill of Health is a mindset full of limiting beliefs. I remember a conversation I overheard once at the gym between a man and a woman. The man said, "When you come to the gym, what do you do?" The woman simply said, "I do both." I knew what she meant, but it still somehow surprised me. She meant that she does both cardio and weights, as if those are the only two options. Many gyms are set up this way. There is cardio equipment on one end, and weights on the other. I grew up with these limited options. Since I wanted to be big and strong, I stayed away from the cardio equipment and focused my attention on lifting weights. When I lifted, I isolated body parts. Monday I did chest and triceps, Tuesday I did back and biceps, Wednesday I did shoulders, Thursday I did legs, and Friday was kind of a day to do whatever I wanted. Usually I rested on weekends to give the muscle fibers a chance to recover. This workout schedule is very common. The reason that it was causing me pain when I did it was because it treats the body as a bunch of separate pieces that have nothing to do with each other. Why are there no other options? We have put limits on our workouts and ourselves. Our bodies were designed to do thousands of different movements. But in a typical gym there are maybe 10-20 different motions that you can do. For thousands and thousands of years, humans have existed in a natural environment. Nature was the expert, forcing people to move in order to survive. Our notion of movement is extremely limiting.

The Treadmill of Health paradigm is not working. Human beings were meant to move, but we don't move enough. Then when we do move, it's not enough to offset the effects of our sedentary lifestyle. There are injuries associated

with people's exercise routines now more than ever because we train some muscles and neglect others, resulting
in imbalance. Hip, knee, and shoulder replacements are
a "normal" part of our modern world. Between 1998 and
2005, the number of total hip replacement surgeries went
from 160,000 to over 230,000 per year (according to the
American Academy of Orthopedic Surgeons). The aver-
age age of clients getting partial hip replacements has gone
from almost 80-years-old to younger than 65-years-old.
Our bodies seem to be breaking down at a record rate and
at a younger age. Are we becoming too frail to function in
our modern world? Have our bodies degenerated so much
that reaching down to pick up a quarter produces the worst
back spasm of our lives? I have a hard time believing
anyone who says that the human body is frail and prone to
breakdown (unfortunately, I have heard many people say
this). This is the same body that survived for millions of
years in the harshest conditions that this world has to offer.
The body is not faulty, it's that we haven't used it properly.

USE IT OR LOSE IT

The human body is an amazing machine. It has the remark-
able ability to adapt to its environment. This adaptation
mechanism was how our ancestors survived such harsh
conditions in the past. We can train our bodies to do almost
anything because our bodies adapt to the environment that
they're placed in. This is why you get bigger when you
lift weights, or why you don't feel good after staring at a
computer all day. Our bodies are literally shaped by the
environment that they're in. We still possess the same
adaptation mechanism of our ancestors, but our bodies are
adapting to a very different environment. We no longer
really need to move. Many of our daily tasks have become
automated. To eat, we only have to walk into a grocery
store, drop some money, and then we're on our way. Humans have never had it so easy. Our ancestors had to find,
kill, or harvest their own food. They didn't sit as much
as we do either. Think of the three major sitting inven-

tions (car, television, computer). All of these have been developed in very recent history. First it was the car, which meant that we didn't have to ride a horse or walk anymore. Then it was the television, which meant we didn't have to talk or move to entertain ourselves anymore. Next came the computer, which meant that we could do massive amounts of "work" without even moving. We have made our lives so much easier, but we are paying the price. Muscles get stronger when they're worked, and weaker when they're not worked. Our muscles atrophy from lack of movement. We don't move enough to keep ourselves healthy, so pain results. Then when we go to move, they are not strong enough to move correctly. We are experiencing chronic movement deprivation. We have introduced a vicious cycle into our society: the less we move, the less we are able to move.

How did our ancestors do it? Before all of our modern conveniences, humans had to work. Our lives are luxurious compared to our forefathers. But our modern conveniences are double-edged swords: they provide us with great ease because there are a lot of things that we no longer need to do, but they are also robbing us of movement. I remember watching a science fiction movie as a kid where the aliens had really big heads to fit their big brains, but their bodies were so frail that they could barely hold up their head. Our reality is not far from this science fiction fantasy. Our lives are devoid of the movements that we need to maintain balance and function. If we want to restore that natural human strength that our ancestors had, we need to get off of the Treadmill of Health.

Until now, human beings have received adequate amounts of movement from their environments. Now we live in a time when we don't have to move. For the first time in history, we must deliberately feed our bodies with proper motions just like we feed ourselves with food and water. We cannot go directly from our desk jobs into a gym, pump out some weights and cardio, and then go home. Our muscles have become imbalanced and weak from all of the inactivity. When we go into the gym, we take in a compromised body. We must restore function before we venture into any other type of activity.

The Treadmill of Health will keep on turning, but we don't have to participate in it. We can reverse the effects of our sedentary lifestyle to enjoy the health we always wanted. The key is to change how we think about movement and exercise. We need to adopt a new paradigm, one that will empower us to live without pain in this automated world.

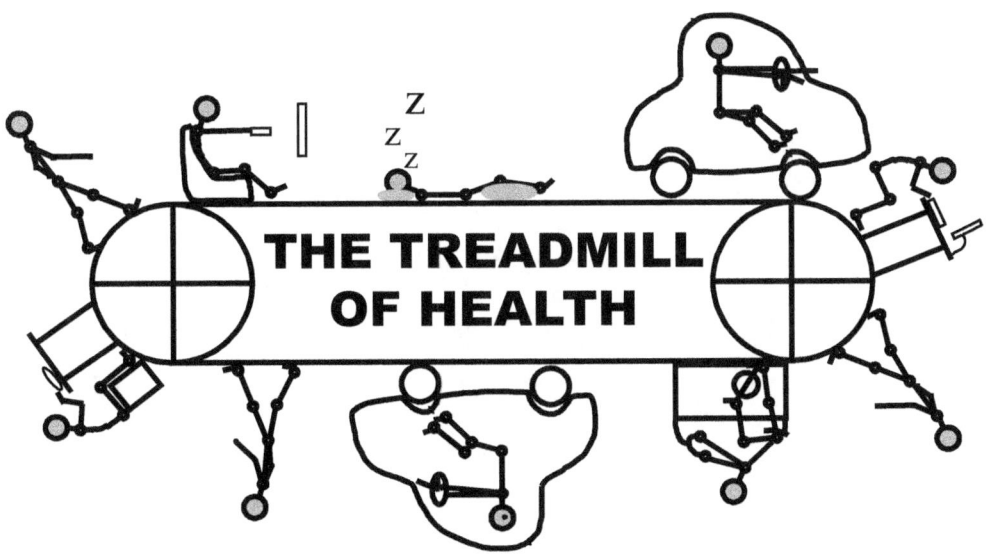

PART TWO

A New Paradigm

THE NEW MEASURING STICK

It is clear that we need to adopt a new way of looking at how we move in our world. We have so many conveniences pulling us toward a motionless life that we need to consciously add more movement. Our new paradigm needs to consider what environment our body would thrive in and what our bodies need. But it also needs to be realistic in seeing that technology is not going away, and therefore we cannot replicate the environment of our ancestors. The solution is not going back to "a simpler time," when everyone picked and hunted their own food. We don't need to change the world that we live in. We need to undo the effects of inactivity, and then introduce functional movements. We must also realize that we don't just need more motion, we need better motion. There is a certain quality of movement that our bodies need to stay healthy. We need to be strong enough not only to function in our environment, but also strong enough to move our bodies without pain or limitation. This type of strength is called functional strength.

Let's get clearer on what functional strength is and how we can develop it in our modern world. The Treadmill of Health uses "maximums" to determine your level of health and fitness. How do we measure functional strength? There is an objective way for us to judge whether we're functional, and that measurement is posture. The lifestyle of our ancestors provided them with enough movement to keep them healthy. This strength was balanced, and this balance manifested itself in their posture. On the other hand, most people in our society are slouching, imbalanced, and not able to control their own bodies the same way that our ancestors could. Posture is merely visual evidence that your body is balanced, front to back, left to right, inside to outside. The measuring stick of function comes in the form of proper posture.

FORM FOLLOWS FUNCTION:
THE PROOF IS IN YOUR POSTURE

Gaining functional strength is what will allow for greater body control and balance. The body's form becomes the way to judge function. "Form follows function" is the case for other objects that exist, too. For example, a bookcase looks the way it looks (form) because its job is to hold and display books (function). A hammer looks the way it looks (form) because its job is to hammer nails (function). If you tried to use a bookcase like a hammer, it wouldn't work. The body also looks a certain way (form) because of how it was designed to function. We were designed to jump, run, climb, crawl, skip, and do a host of other activities without experiencing pain or difficulty. When our bodies don't get their daily dose of movement, function begins to break down. When function breaks down, our posture (form) becomes compromised. At this point, it's a downward cycle. When the body is not functional, trying to do even basic movements will lead to a change in form. When this change occurs, we call it compensation. The body cannot do the movement the way that it was designed to, so it compensates to get it done. These compensations are readily visible to observers. By watching the body's form, we can judge how functional it is.

Based on the relationship between form and function, we can develop a definition of functional strength. Our working definition of functional strength will simply be: "One's ability to execute a movement with the proper form, or posture." The less your body compensates, the more functional you are and vice versa. When walking, a limp is evidence of a dysfunctional body. One part is not able to do its job, so you have to change your entire body's mechanics in order to walk. If you knew what to look for, you could watch anybody do anything and would be able to judge how functional he or she is. Whether that's reaching overhead to get a dish from the kitchen cabinet, walking up stairs, or even just standing still, you can tell a lot about a person's level of function by watching their form. Maybe they have to fling their knee out to the side before they step up, or perhaps their torso has to rotate to the side for them to get their arm over their head. These are correctable compensations, just evidence of a muscular imbalance. If you know what to look for, you can spot these compensations easily. Some people's shoulders round forward, one hip may be rotated in front of the other, or the feet could be turned out. These compensations give us the visual feedback that we are not functional. The posture test applies whether you're 10 or 110. The benefit of functional strength over maximum strength is that the more functional you get, the less pain you have and the less likely you are to injure yourself. You also gain more body control, which means you become a better athlete. As your posture im-

26

proves, your body achieves a natural balance. Gaining functional strength will enable us to go through our lives without compensations, and therefore without pain or limitation.

We've talked about form, function, and compensations. But how do we know what the form is supposed to look like? What are the specific landmarks on the body that we should look at? The good news is that you don't have to be an anatomy expert to understand this. The body's eight load-bearing joints and the curve of the spine will show us how functional somebody is. These include your two shoulders, two hips, two knees, and two ankles. From the side, your spine should have a slight "S" curve and you should be able to draw a vertical line up from the ankle that intersects the middle of the knee, hip, and shoulder on the same side. From the front and back views, your body should form a grid, a series of 90-degree angles from the ankles all the way up to the shoulders. This basic position allows for proper movement of the entire body. It is called Human Design Posture. Function does not depend on how big your muscles are. It can be restored regardless of age or ability. This basic body position is how we should be as humans, it is our birthright. With this position as the measuring stick, we don't need to worry about how big the muscles are, how much you can bench press, or your VO2 max. This position tells us how functional you are. This is the foundation of all movement.

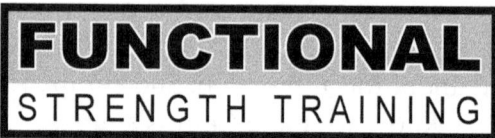

Human Design Posture

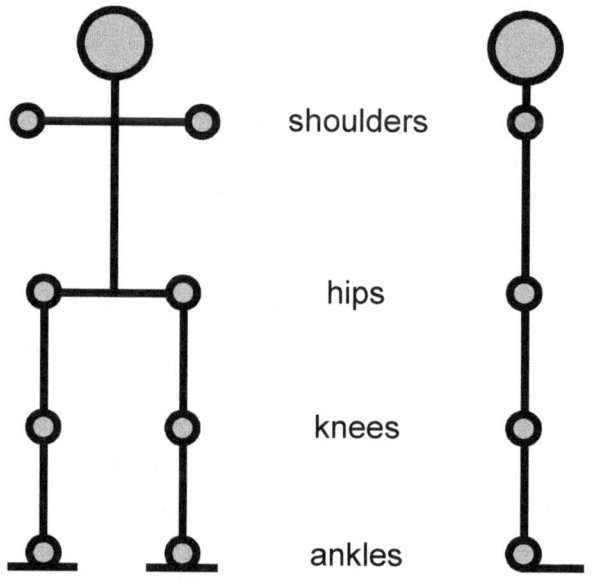

shoulders

hips

knees

ankles

Left and right sides should be balanced, as well as front and back. This balance should be effortless.

www.FSTworkout.com

FUNCTION IS FOUNDATIONAL

If a human being were a skyscraper, functional strength
would be the concrete foundation and the steel beams
that run throughout the structure. They keep the building
straight and vertical. This foundation is what the engineers
and architects care about. The rest is secondary. If this
basic foundation is flawed, it doesn't matter what else you
put on the outside, the building is doomed. It will succumb
to the first major earthquake, flood, or harsh winds. If the
foundation is solid, it will withstand the natural disasters
unharmed. The worst disaster could break the windows
and rip off the roof, but if that building has a solid foundation it will still stand. Like a building's foundation, functional strength is our body's foundation.

Similar to the steel beams of a high-rise, the body has its
own internal stabilization system. It's not made of steel or
concrete, it consists of muscles. But the muscles that keep

your body in a certain position are deep. They are intrinsic, sitting close to the bones. Your body keeps its vertical alignment through a balanced tension relationship of these muscles that run throughout your body. These muscles are not big and bulky, they are underlying. When you lift a lot of weight, they are not doing the lifting, they are stabilizing the joints. You've probably heard a lot of talk about "core" muscles. These muscles are your core. They are responsible for the position of your body and they have nothing to do with how "buff" you are. Restoring our Human Design Posture restores our body's foundation, or core.

GRAVITY AND GAIT

Our bodies have adapted to their surroundings for millions
of years. One very basic law exists regardless of where you
live or where your ancestors originated. Gravity. Gravity
is so essential to proper function that I cannot afford to skip
it. Our bodies were designed to function in an environment
that has a gravitational pull in it. How do I know this?
Have you ever seen video of astronauts after they return
from space? Spending just a month in space deprives
them of so much good gravity that they can barely stand
up on earth. Just like movement, gravity is essential for
our bodies. So why am I even telling you this? Most of
us don't think about venturing into space. It's likely that
you're never going to try to escape to the moon. Gravity
is not something that we have much of a choice over. But
we can change gravity in ways we don't really think about.
Think about the person who decides to work out in a pool
from now on because their joints hurt. The pool workouts

feel good because there is no pounding on the joints. There is nothing wrong with pool workouts, but you should not use them as the only place you move. Although many swimmers are very strong, the deep postural muscles are not necessarily holding the body where it needs to be. If we're in pain, working out in a pool may be good for a while. But we must know that instead of hiding from injuries by creating a weight-less environment, we need to train our bodies to be functional in gravity. This is the environment that our bodies were designed to be in, and the environment that we get the most benefits from. We need to re-educate our bodies on how to best function in gravity. This happens when our posture and function have been restored.

The most basic functional movement for a human being is walking, or gait. Have you ever noticed how you can identify most people by how they walk? Everyone seems to have a signature when it comes to his or her specific gait pattern. The reason for this is that each person's walk is the visual manifestation of how his or her muscles are functioning. Changing how their muscles work would change their walk. Here's an example: have you ever mimicked somebody's walk for a long period of time? Doesn't your body begin to feel different? If you walked pigeon-toed all day (toes pointed in toward each other), you would begin to feel different muscles working to keep you in that position. You may even feel pain. The reason why some people walk pigeon-toed naturally and others don't is because of a different relationship among their muscles. People have different compensation patterns because of different lifestyles, which result in different aches and pains. You can discover a lot about a person's functional ability from their gait.

HOW MUSCLES MOVE BONES

At this point, it would help for us to establish an understanding of how posture can be changed. We will only need a basic understanding of how muscles and bones work. Posture and function are not complicated, so you don't need any background to understand it. Like I said in the Introduction, I could explain this to a six-year-old and they would understand it. The following pages are simplified representations of what happens in your body. If this were all that you read, you would have more knowledge about the dynamics of posture than if you were to memorize the name of every muscle in the body.

To understand posture, you need to understand how muscles move bones. Every muscle in your body connects two or more bones together. Imagine that the muscles are glued to bones at both ends. It's like cutting a rubber band, and then connecting each end to a different Popsicle stick.

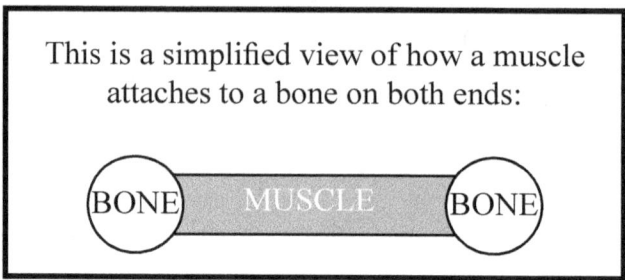

The rubber band represents a muscle, and the two Popsicle sticks represent bones. There are hundreds of these connections throughout your entire body, which combine to form the structure of the human body. But for the sake of understanding, let's just focus on the function of a single muscle, attached to two bones.

Muscles contract to bring those bones closer to each other. When muscles relax, the bones move away from each other. To see an example, bend your elbow to bring your hand closer to your shoulder. Now lower it down. Your bicep contracted to bring the hand up, and relaxed to bring your hand down. When you contracted your muscle, you produced tension, which shortened your muscle. When you relaxed the muscle, the tension went away and the muscle lengthened.

Each muscle in our bodies has a specific range of motion. This range represents how far your muscle can stretch and contract comfortably. When your arm is completely straight, your bicep is at its longest comfortable position, which signifies one end of its range of motion. When you bend your elbow to bring your hand toward your shoulder, the bicep shortens. When you squeeze the bicep as hard as you can, you put it in its shortest position. This muscle length signifies the other end of its range of motion. There is a limit to how long each muscle should get and how short each muscle should get. For example, if you were to hyperextend your elbow, your bicep would lengthen past its desired range of motion. A muscle's range of motion refers to how much that muscle can be stretched and contracted comfortably.

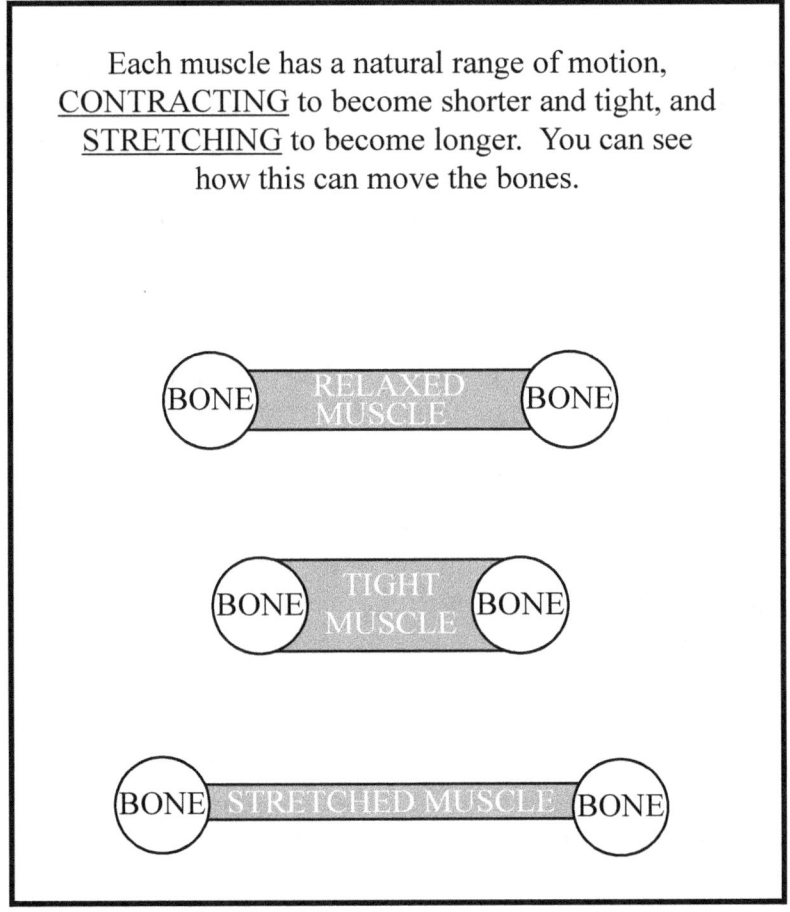

Each muscle has a natural range of motion, CONTRACTING to become shorter and tight, and STRETCHING to become longer. You can see how this can move the bones.

Every muscle also has a desired resting position. This position is the length of the muscle when it is relaxed. It's the position that it returns to when you are not contracting or stretching that particular muscle. If you had a rubber band lying on the table, it would naturally be in its resting position. If you stretched that rubber band around the circumference of a football, it would get longer. But if you took it off of the football, it would return to its resting position. If you kept the rubber band on that football too long, then it may never return to its resting position. It has become too stretched, and therefore too long. This is similar to what happens in your body. If you keep a muscle too stretched or too tight for too long, then it will begin to shift its resting position. Since it is the job of muscles to move bones, then the bones will shift their positions. Posture will become compromised because the muscles no longer hold the bones where they should be. The one advantage that human beings have over rubber bands is that we can correct our imbalances. That rubber band will probably never return to its desired length, but we can return our muscles to their optimal length, and therefore optimal function. We do this by lengthening the contracted muscles and shortening the stretched muscles. Once every muscle is returned to its desired resting position, proper posture and function have been restored, and we enjoy all of the benefits our bodies have to offer us. This is the basic concept of posture. Once you understand this concept, you've got it.

Let's recap all of our vocabulary words. Connecting two bones, you have a muscle. This connection looks like a rubber band glued to two Popsicle sticks. This muscle contracts and shortens to move these bones closer together, then relaxes and lengthens to move them farther apart. The distance that this muscle travels between the shortest position and the longest position is its range of motion. Every muscle has a resting position, which is the length that it naturally returns to when it's not moving.

How does a change in one muscle's length affect other muscles? When we contract our muscles, those muscle contractions don't occur in isolation. Each time one muscle contracts, its opposite muscle relaxes. This is how we can affect more than just the muscle being contracted. Let's go back to the example of the bicep. The bicep's opposing muscle is the tricep. So when the bicep shortens, the tricep lengthens, and vice versa. Each muscle is designed to be at a certain length when compared to the other muscles. If the lengths are distorted, you will see it in your posture (remember, form follows function). For example, imagine

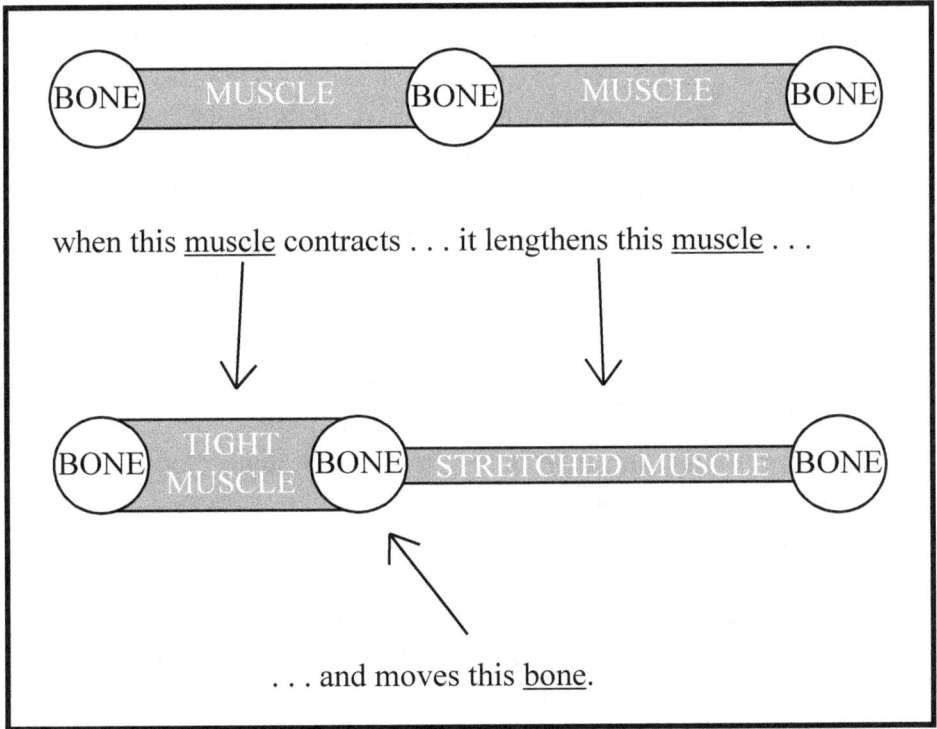

your biceps were really tight and short in their resting position. This would mean that your triceps would be lengthened in their resting position. Now they are both in positions where they cannot function optimally. And what's worse, your body feels like this is the normal position to be in, so your concept of "neutral" is way off. Your body has changed its resting position. In this scenario, your elbows would always be bent. You would feel like that was natural.

Let's go back to the above scenario of the tight biceps. Imagine that you were reading this and you just realized that you have tight biceps. You might try to lock out your arms when you walk because you know that that's how it's supposed to be. But this would be wrong. "Resting position" applies to how our muscles hold the bones if we aren't trying to force it. It's important to know that proper posture is natural. When the body is balanced, it just happens. It is not something that you have to think about all day long. Forcing "good posture" is no better than having bad posture. More often than not, when someone forces their posture, they are really just pulling their shoulders back. Doing this does not address the hundreds of other muscles that are off. Posture is evidence of your muscle balance, and cannot be forced.

Re-read the previous few paragraphs and look at the pictures as many times as you need to grasp it. Once you understand these concepts, you understand posture. That's it. It really is that simple. You don't need to memorize the 600+ muscles in the body. This basic concept will allow you to understand how the position of your body can be changed. Understanding how one muscle works will carry over into an understanding of how the entire body works.

HOW MUSCLES MOVE BONES

It is not about memorization, it is more conceptual than anything else. Next we'll dive into how these basic concepts manifest in your body in a more realistic example of a common compensation.

A basic example of muscles working in pairs and how it affects other muscles:

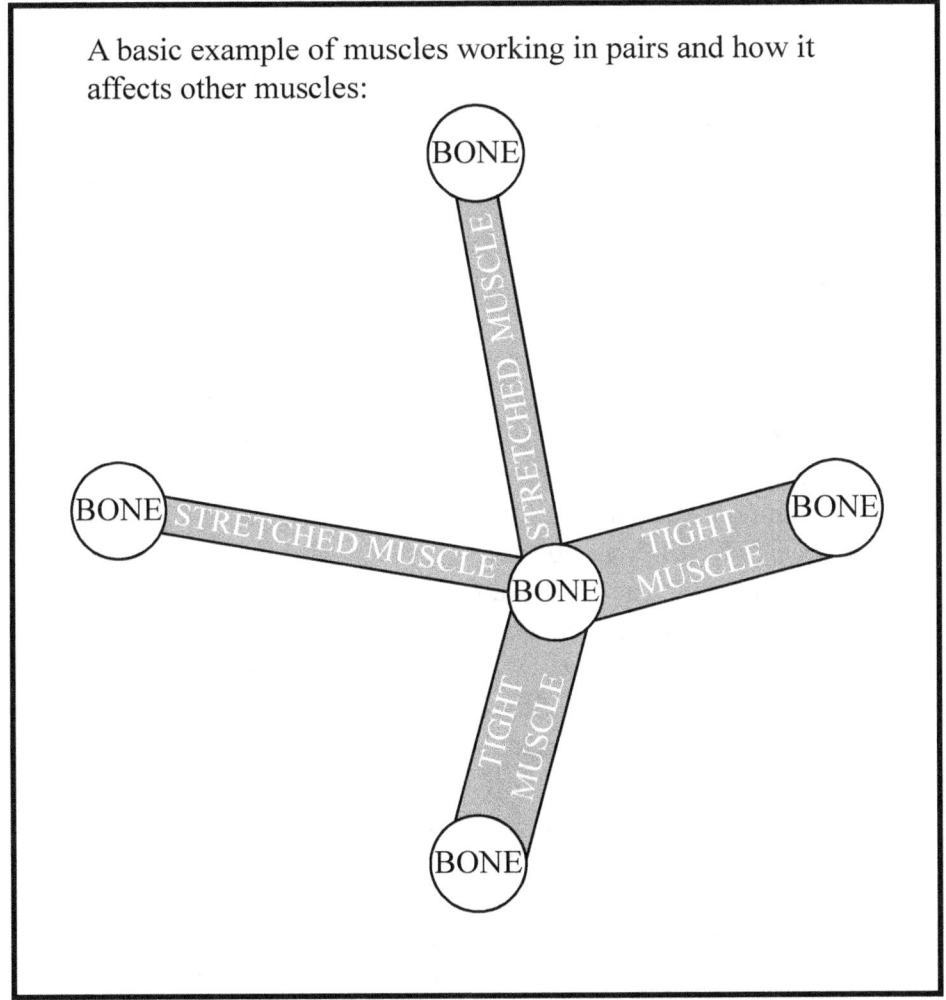

A COMMON COMPENSATION

In our society, we sit a lot. How do our bodies respond to sitting? What effect does this have on the resting position of our muscles? Let's look at how a group of compensations can result from sitting too much. When you sit, you are basically folding your body 90-degrees from the hip. The direction of this fold is considered "flexion." Remember that every muscle attaches to bones and pulls them toward each other. The muscles that we're going to focus on right now are the hip flexors. These muscles are located in the front of the hip and attach from the top of the leg to the lower back. When you are standing and you raise your knee straight up you are using these muscles. They are called your hip flexors, because simply, they flex the hip. When you sit, your hip flexors are put into a shortened position. Prolonged sitting will change the resting length of the hip flexors. Your body now thinks that this shortened position is normal. It will initiate every move-

40

ment from this shortened position. Now, go to stand up with your short hip flexors and we have a problem. Your body has to compensate for the hip flexors's inability to reach its full length. One common compensation is the spine gets pulled out of its normal position to accommodate the tight hip. When this happens, this places pressure on your lower back. You have just completely altered where the bones, muscles, and nerves are supposed to be. This compensation works its way up and down the body. Every muscle has to adjust itself to compensate for the change in the hips and back. The upper spine will change to offset the big arch in the lower back. The result is a shift away from a subtle spinal "S" curve, into an exaggerated curve. This affects the neck and shoulders, which will now have to reposition to compensate for the need for balance. Your body wants to stay standing, and it won't let the hip flexors ruin that. It will find a way to stand even though it is not the best way. The compensation pattern will run down the legs too. The thigh and hamstring muscles connect to the pelvis, which has been altered from the constant sitting. These two muscle groups also connect down to the knee. Because they have to change their resting lengths the knees will move. The feet follow in what becomes an overflow of compensations. Now, because of the altered resting position of everything, new compensations begin to develop in response to the first group of compensations. Now you've just stacked another layer of faulty movements on top of the old one. If you took this body to the gym and pumped out some reps on the bench press, you could be setting yourself up for injury. Unless these postural imbalances are addressed before you begin an activity, your body will compensate in that activity. When we correct the compensation, your body's resting position is restored, and every muscle can work the way it was designed to work.

To make this correction, we cannot focus on correcting one muscle at a time. When we restore functional movements, all of the muscles will follow.

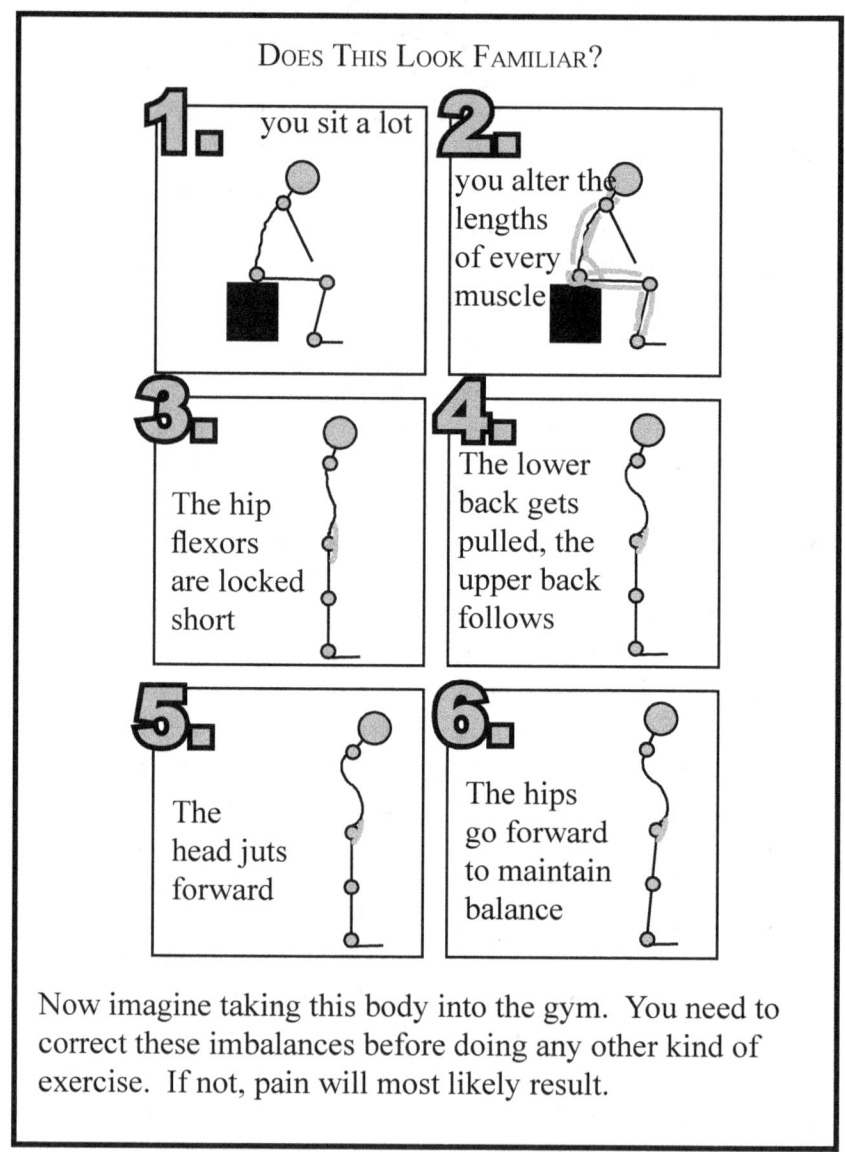

DOES THIS LOOK FAMILIAR?

1. you sit a lot

2. you alter the lengths of every muscle

3. The hip flexors are locked short

4. The lower back gets pulled, the upper back follows

5. The head juts forward

6. The hips go forward to maintain balance

Now imagine taking this body into the gym. You need to correct these imbalances before doing any other kind of exercise. If not, pain will most likely result.

THINK "MOVEMENTS" NOT "MUSCLES"

Once you understand the concept that "muscles move bones," you can put muscles out of your head. What I mean by that is that when your posture is off, it is not the responsibility of just one muscle. Every muscle is off. We need to focus on functional movements to re-establish our function. The body works as one unit. Each part helps to balance, stabilize, and assist other parts of the body. If one part of the body is not stable or has a faulty range of motion, then the rest of the body must compensate for that dysfunction. Proper movements need to be emphasized if we hope to eliminate the compensation patterns that have developed in the body. We must always see the body as one unit. For example, when we're doing an exercise where there is shoulder movement, we're still aware of the position of the feet, legs, hips, and spine. Changing one piece of that puzzle can change the entire outcome of the exercise.

43

Let's look at a specific example of the body working as one unit. When you go to step off of a curb to cross the street, your body must be able to properly transfer weight to one leg while extending the other. The stabilizing leg must control the forces that are acting on your body and simultaneously accept your entire body weight. As the legs are doing this, it's sending a force up the torso, which the back and abs must stabilize so that you don't fall over. That's a lot to do in a short amount of time! If you are dysfunctional, this motion will become compromised, resulting in a lack of balance, slow movements, or pain. Because of the faulty range of motion and resting position, every muscle changes how it works, and the entire body changes how it moves.

In the Introduction, when I was trying to get myself out of pain, I mentioned that stretching didn't work. Then later in the book I wrote that restoring posture is a combination of stretching tight muscles and shortening your stretched muscles. I know that these statements may seem to contradict each other, but let me show you how they don't. Many people in our society complain of having tight hamstrings (I used to be one of them). They stretch and stretch, but the hamstrings don't seem to be loosening up. If we were to take a picture of that person standing from the side view, most likely we would see that their hips are in front of the gravity line (If we drew a line straight up from the person's ankle, this would be called the "gravity line"). The gravity line is where your 8 load-bearing joints should sit in order to restore proper balance. The reason the person's hamstrings feel tight is because the pelvis is out of position. So they could stretch their hamstrings all day, but until they change where the hips and pelvis are naturally positioned, their tightness will remain. It's not just about stretching. Re-positioning the bones and joints are key.

THINK "MOVEMENTS" NOT "MUSCLES"

It is not the job of any one muscle to walk, jump, run, skip, or climb. We perform these motions using a combination of muscles and forces. We must focus on natural, functional movements that emphasize the body's specific movement requirements. As we gain more functional strength, we are better able to use the body as one unit the way it was intended. We are better able to function in our environment without limitations that result from improper training, sitting, or injury. With this new understanding of movement, we can see that we don't need to fall victim to injuries or even minor discomfort. We can re-establish our body's innate functional ability regardless of age, size, gender, or ability. Our bodies were meant to move freely without compensation. Our society's current paradigm, The Treadmill of Health, is not providing us adequate movement to keep us functional. But it's never too late to get it back.

PART THREE

FUNCTIONAL STRENGTH TRAINING

THE PROCESS

Functional Strength Training (FST) uses systematic tech-
niques to improve your posture. All of our trainers are up
to date on the current certifications and information. We
use this knowledge to create drastic changes in our clients'
functional strength. Our goal is to return your body to
Human Design Posture through functional movements that
treat the body as a unit. We look at your posture (form)
and determine your level of function. Once we do this,
your body is able to benefit from the most basic premise
of exercise: the body is changeable. Many people feel
like they can move easier. Motion doesn't feel so forced.
Many notice an increase in balance and athleticism. Often,
morning aches and pains subside. The more functional you
get, the better you feel in your own skin. But you must
be committed. It helps when you find that spark inside of
yourself. Get absolutely fed up with even low-level pains.
If you fully commit yourself, you will feel the difference

very quickly. Most people feel like they're lighter and taller from just one session. From that point, you need to re-enforce the positive changes daily. Working together, we can build you a program that corrects your dysfunctions and compensations and fits into your life.

As you progress with the program, not only will you feel better but you'll also have visual proof that you are getting more functional because we gauge your progress with posture photos. Since form follows function, your posture will continue to improve, as you get more functional. That feedback helps to keep you motivated and directed toward your goal. It also helps us to determine how your body is compensating so that we can help you return to your Human Design Posture.

FST is located in Santa Clara, California. We see clients in our studio throughout the day, weekends too. We can help whether you're in our geographic area or not. Since we can judge how functional you are by looking at your standing posture, we offer Online Posture Alignment Therapy. To participate in this program, all you have to do is send us four pictures of yourself (standing position front, back, left, and right). From those pictures, we can get an idea of what your particular compensations are. Once we have gathered all the information that we need, we begin to implement a series of corrective exercises that are designed for you. It takes constant communication, whether in-studio or online, so that we can monitor your form and address any questions you have in the process. We have had tremendous success both in-studio and online. Visit www.FSTworkout.com/online.html for specific information about our Online Posture Therapy Program.

SOME MORE BENEFITS OF
PROPER FUNCTION

I've seen some incredible things as a Posture Alignment Specialist. I have several clients who don't even break a sweat during "workouts." Yet, despite this, they have lost inches from their legs, hips, and stomachs. Their workouts include relatively easy exercises to re-introduce lost ranges of motion. Because of the balancing nature of the workouts, they have reshaped their bodies, and dropped several sizes. Remember, "no pain, no gain" is out. Restoring proper function allowed these people to change their bodies without feeling deprived from cutting calories and without doing excessive amounts of "cardio."

There are other benefits to being functional that at first glance may seem unrelated to exercise. For example, digestion can improve because of a change in posture. The digestive system is a series of tubes that course through your torso area. If your spine, ribs, and torso are out of

alignment, then this will change the position of the digestive system as well. This applies to all organs in your chest
cavity. The organs are designed to function in a certain
position. Once the proper position is restored, then internal
organs can function properly as well. Many clients experience this result as they get functional.

I can't forget the cosmetic results of training this way.
When you're functional, you are lean and balanced. All
muscles look properly proportioned. When someone sees a
functional person, they say things like, "that's how a person
is supposed to look." Functional strength is not distorted or
bulky, but rather it is balanced and natural looking. Since
you are not isolating specific muscles, all of your muscles
are strong. You're just the right proportion for your particular body type.

WHY SETTLE FOR LESS THAN
YOU DESERVE?

Exercise is about transformation. It's about knowing that the way things have been is not necessarily the way they always have to be. The Treadmill of Health thinks that our muscle aches and pains are a natural part of life. We forget about being able to go all day long without a backache. Many gym-goers exercise for 30 minutes and get tired. They wonder what happened. Where did it go? Functional strength is about bringing "it" back again. FST brings you back to your body, and reintroduces you to something that has always been inside of you. We do not create it for you. You reconnect to where you came from, that flexible body that you had as a child. Turning back the clock is easier than you think. Trust me, I've done it.

MOTIVATION FOR THE JOURNEY

"How long will this take?" This is probably the most common question that I hear as a trainer. Understandably, people want to know how long it will be before they can call themselves "functional." There is no doubt that if you want to permanently correct your alignment and increase your function you will need long-term sustained effort. It demands time and attention everyday. You will encounter times when you are not seeing the results that you want. Other times, you will feel like a new person everyday. It's not always a straight climb to the top of the mountain, but never give up. There are bumps as well as straight climbs, ups as well as downs. If you stay consistent doing your daily functional routine, your progress will look much like the stock market graph, there are highs and lows but if you zoom out enough it tends to go up. You must take the long view approach if you desire to be successful. It takes both daily attention and long-term evaluation. Every detail must be focused on, but when evaluating progress use weeks and months. Nothing worthwhile is ever quick. The results that you want are waiting for you, and they are incredible.

The speed that you travel depends a lot on you. How focused are you? How is your form when you do the exercises? How much time do you spend daily? How many days a week do you do the exercises? Do you rush through them or are you deliberate? How long have you been doing alignment exercises? If you have had chronic pain, don't expect it to go away with one hour once or twice a week. It takes a huge commitment, and it must be done daily. Do whatever works for you to keep your motivation levels high. Listen to tapes, watch inspirational videos, and read about successful people. It may also help to re-read this book once a month or so. It's a quick read, and it will keep you in touch with why you're doing this. This is your functional journey.

With persistence and patience, we can move away from the outdated Treadmill of Health paradigm, and toward a more balanced view of health. At FST we are excited to be a part of that change. We are committed to empowering clients to make profound changes in their lives. Once committed to the process, you will sail through. If you don't commit, and you only do your exercises sometimes, you will not see much of a change. If you understand what's at stake, you will get the motivation you need. Remember those hip replacement statistics? Until our society gets more functional, I'm afraid those statistics will only get worse. We must re-gain control over our health. You have the chance to change your life. That should excite you.

I encourage you to get in touch with the reasons why you

want to get functional. Once you have those, the rest comes naturally. Ask yourself "why?" Why did you pick up this book? Why are you interested in this? Why do you want to become functional? How badly do you want to change? I know that there is a reason that you are reading this. I hit a point in my life where I had zero tolerance for pain. Once that happened, the rest was easier. The hard part was getting to that point. The key is to raise your standards. Don't accept that you have to live in pain for the rest of your life. You can change your body, and the time to do that is now. It's not rocket science, it's just simple exercises that restore the balance that is lost throughout our motionless days. Don't settle for less than you deserve.

Most likely you have a favorite sport or activity that you want to start doing again. I encourage you to use this as motivation. As I said before, function is foundational. Functional strength will be the foundation to whatever you want to do. At FST, we don't expect to keep training a client forever. You will get to the point where your functional ability and posture are good. Then you become like a bird leaving the nest. You continue to do your exercises before and after your activities, and it keeps you out of pain. This type of training was designed to empower you to take control over your own health. You use this information how you want. My job is merely to show you another way, and help you get functional. Once you're functional, if you want to stick around FST and take a small group class, that's great. If you want to participate in our camps, all the better. But you won't have to use FST as a crutch. You can do whatever you want. Function will free your body to move however you feel inspired to move. Most importantly, you will have the tools to keep yourself functional in this motionless world.

DEAR READER,

You may have noticed that there are not exercises in this book. That was done deliberately for two reasons. First, I firmly believe that you should be looked at and given a set of exercises that is customized to you, even if you only get that done one time. Once is better than none at all. If you live outside of the Bay Area, I strongly encourage you to try our Online Posture Alignment Therapy program. It is very easy to do, and you are still working with a real person, through e-mail communication. The second reason I haven't put exercises in this book is because websites are easier to update than books are. I have created a page on my website exclusively for people who read the book. This site will keep you up to date on the newest that we have to offer. Visit
www.FSTworkout.com/FunctionalStrengthBook.html
to visit that page directly. It has generalized posture exercises and routines that you can try to get a feel for what it's all about. After doing the general routine for a while, you will be ready for your own.

Education is very important to me. The FST website has even more resources to help you understand the importance of posture and function. I want to keep the lines of communication open, so feel free to contact me with any questions, comments, or concerns that you may have. I want to be of service any way that I can, so I truly welcome your comments. I wish you the very best in your journey toward functional strength, and I look forward to working with you soon.

In Health,

Chris Janke

Check out other educational products at:

www.FSTworkout.com